Medicinal Plants

Learn The Basic Beginner Benefits Of These Top Medicinal Plants For Healing Your Self Naturally With Natural Medicinal Plants

Table Of Contents

Introduction

Why I Wrote This Book

What You Should Know Before Reading This Book

Chapter 1 : Garlic

Chapter 2 : Cloves

Chapter 3 : Peppermint

Chapter 4 : Aloe Vera

Chapter 5 : Turmeric

Chapter 6 :Cardamom

Conclusion

Disclaimer

The information provided in this book is designed to provide helpful information on the subjects discussed. This book is not meant to be used, nor should it be used, to diagnose or treat any medical condition. For diagnosis or treatment of any medical problem, consult your own physician. The publisher and author are not responsible for any specific health or allergy needs that may require medical supervision and are not liable for any damages or negative consequences from any treatment, action, application or preparation, to any person reading or following the information in this book. Any references included are provided for informational purposes only and do not constitute endorsement of any websites or other sources. Readers should be aware that any websites listed in this book may change.

Introduction

Every once in a while it can become very difficult for us to trust the medical industry when we find ourselves in any kind of medicinal distress. Because of the unsavory ways people within the medical and pharmaceutical industry, it can be extremely difficult for us to get answers when we need them and solutions to problems rather than temporary fixes. If you have a hard time trusting the medical industry, you are definitely not alone. All of us have a hard time at some point in our lives, especially once we realize that being said is profitable to certain types of people. And these people are the ones in charge of helping us when we need it the most.

Too many times we find ourselves challenged by illnesses and bad health. Because of the way that the world works, many of the foods that we are actually toxic to us and can cause major problems in our bodies. If we are not able to address these problems and work toward positive solutions rather than temporary solutions that can end up causing more issues with their side effects, then we may end up finding ourselves with too many chemicals in the body and not feeling very happy to be guinea pigs of experimental medicines that are just out to make the people in the pharmaceutical industry a lot of money.

Overall, it can be very discouraging to see that the medical industry profits from our pain, and because of this more and more people have become tempted to investigate the benefits of medicinal plants. Many of these plants have been proven time and time again to help the body to reduce inflammation, fight off bacteria and diseases, and even to fight cancer. If you are interested in finding out how these plants can heal you, starting now, and help to prevent further medical issues within you further on down the road, this is the book for you.

Reading about medicinal plants may be the most responsible thing you have ever done for your health, and unfortunately many companies are out there in the world trying to keep their hands in the pockets of oblivious consumers, who are willing to eat terrible foods and be treated by terrible medicines when they are no longer being nourished by their foods, but rather, poisoned by them.

Why I Wrote This Book

I wrote this book because I am worried about the people in the world. It is not fair for all of us to have to live in fear of the things we eat and the medicines that we use to treat ourselves and we are ill. Nobody should have to worry about whether or not our doctors are giving us something that they know may not help us. Medicines that have way too many side effects are dangerous, and I resent being used as a guinea pig and medical experimentation. I don't think it's fair for everybody to have their good bacteria wiped out by antibiotics that are extremely unhealthy for the body as a whole. These antibiotics can even cause severe yeast infections and many people, and other dangerous side effects that can impair us for the rest of our lives.

The damage that is done by experimental medicine is infinite. These are consumed by us and then flushed out of bodies, put into the water supply and into the oceans and rivers where marine life lives and is affected by them as well. We are not the only ones who are being poisoned by these dangerous and irresponsible drugs, there are many plants and Marine animals out there that are negatively impacted by our overdependence on chemical pharmaceuticals. These chemicals make it into their homes and disrupt their lives, leading to deformities and difficulties with being in their environment and habitats.

We all deserve somewhere safe and desirable to live, somewhere that is natural and will not harm us more than helps us. Nobody should be harmed by these terrible things, and yet so many people are. Even though it is experimental, it is still prescribed as if they know that we will not be affected negatively by it. The lawsuits that they are faced with later on down the line seem to be nothing when compared to the billions of dollars that they make from poisoning the overall population with their experimental drugs.

If you want to make sure that you and your family are safe from the dangerous side effects of experimental drugs and modern chemical pharmaceuticals, medicinal plants for beginners is an incredible idea. This basic guide will show you all the ways that medicinal plants can benefit you and your family, and prevent you from getting sick. Ultimately, this will keep you out of the hospital and away from even more dangerous chemical cocktails that could harm us later on down the line.

What You Need To Know Before Reading This Book

Before you read this book , it is important to remember that everybody may have different reactions to different plants. We all may be vulnerable to specific allergies that may or may not pertain to us, and so using new plants for medicinal purposes should always be approached with caution when you are attempting to experiment with new medicinal plants. You can approach the use of a new plant is by simply trying to use a spot test or only ingesting a little bit of each. It can be dangerous for you to try using medicinal plant you've never used before, especially when you don't know whether or not you will have an adverse reaction to it.

Make sure that you have some kind of allergy medicine on hand, such as Benadryl or an epi-pen at the time of your experiment. Never ingest too much at first, simply ingest a small amount before you attempt to take a large amount for your symptoms. Our tolerance for different foods is always different, and you should always make sure that you are able to make decisions for your body that are going to benefit yourself rather than to harm yourself. Always approach a new food of caution, and don't be silly if one food doesn't work for you. That doesn't mean that other foods might not leader in the future.

It is important to keep an open mind whenever you embark upon a journey when dealing with medicinal plants. Some of these things have been used for centuries, and you should try and understand that there is wisdom and things even have not been scientifically proven. Fortunately, most of these plants have been scientifically tested and proven to have medicinal benefits for the body, which is why they are included in this book. Make sure that you approach each of these caution if you have never tried them before, and more than anything, trying to remember that you do not have to go to the hospital every time you are sick, you can always try and rebalance your own body without the use of chemical drugs that may end up harming you further on down the line.

Chapter 1: Garlic

Most of us can either leave it, because of its strong flavor and its tendency to make our breath smelled very unique. However, garlic has been able to aid the body in healing for centuries, and many people have used it over the years to treat everything from vampires to colds. Garlic is extremely beneficial if you are attempting to detoxify the body and find toxins so that you can lose weight and get rid of the bacteria and germs that can cause many different disorders.

Garlic is also very nutritious and can help to remove the heavy metals in the body that can lead to extreme bouts of illness later on down the line in your life, such as dementia and Alzheimer's. These neurological disorders are caused by toxins that had escaped into the bloodstream and made it into the brain, and their collection here can cause many neurological disorders. Garlic can help to prevent disease as well as cure it.

Not only that, but it can help to boost the immune system and help us to prevent everything from the common cold to yeast infections. Everybody has a great story to tell about garlic when the user as a healing medicinal plant, and it is even easy to grow it for yourself. Don't be deterred by its bad reputation, garlic is actually one of the most beneficial plants that are widely available today. Don't be scared away by the bad breath, your health is a lot more important than something so superficial.

Chapter 2: Cloves

Close something used for a long time, particularly in the treatment of oral problems. Clothes can help to numb the guns and keep everybody healthier in their mouths. The mouth is an epicenter for bacteria, and if your mouth is not clean and healthy, it can cause more problems in your health than you realize. Cloves been used for a long time, particularly in India with the healing art of Ayurveda. Their miraculous benefits can help us to stay strong and even with a way any problems that we might face with the flu virus.

You can even use clove on extra wounds, to treat and dress them easily. It helps to kill germs and bacteria, and can provide relief to the area particularly by numbing it and preventing us from feeling negative and painful emotions. They also cannot your teeth if you have a toothache, which can be one of the most painful afflictions there are. Clove oil is antibacterial and can help us to fight away germs and when they are used in moderation can change our lives.

Chapter 3: Peppermint

Peppermint has been known for centuries for its healing properties, and can allow us to stay healthy for a long time. It circulates blood, increasing blood flow and promoting good health. With peppermint's help, we can begin to treat many afflictions and avoid many others. It is refreshing and tasty, and can help us in many ways.

Peppermint is particularly beneficial if you suffer from issues with digestion. A systemic's and gastrointestinal diseases can cause us to have many problems. If we are suffering from these kinds of issues, it can be very uncomfortable and discomfort can lead us to being cranky and grumpy throughout the day. We have an issue or a bug in our digestive tract, has material properties that can suit these issues. It is soothing to the body and can prevent stomachaches and cure them. It is also beneficial in treating motion sickness and any other type of nausea.

Peppermint is also particularly beneficial when it comes to headaches. All of us seem to be stressed out in this modern day and age, and because of the stress it can cause a lot of tension headaches. Our jobs are very stressful, and surviving in this society can be very difficult. Fortunately for you, peppermint is one of the most healing medicinal plants there are, particularly if you are just a beginner trying to get your feet wet with healing medicinal plants.

Chapter 4: Aloe Vera

Have you ever had a sunburn? Chances are you have. Most of the time, if we had sunburns, the first thing that we do is turn to our aloe their gel. Most of us don't really think about where our aloe vera gel comes from. All we know is that it is in a lot of many different types of cleansers and emotions, because of claims to helping the body and soothing the skin. Have you ever thought to consider where these claims come from?

You have, you probably figured out aloe vera gel comes from the elevator plant, which is relatively common. It's a particularly easy plant to grow, and because of this it is commonly found throughout the world. Aloe vera gel has been used for centuries for helping to soothe and provide relief from other brands. Aloe also help to promote good blood flow and is able to bind up a lot of toxins and free radicals so that they do not make it into our bloodstream and cause us to suffer from needless ailments in the future, such as dementia and Alzheimer's.

Because of this, it can also be said that aloe vera can help us to eliminate way, because of its ability to find toxins in the body and keep us healthy for a long time. It prevents diseases because it's able to work as an antibiotic and find out terrible toxins that can cause major illness. It's a very cleansing and detoxifying agent that can help not only to cure our illnesses to prevent them as well, so you should not ever have to go to the doctor if you are able to keep your body naturally balanced using aloe vera gel and other medicinal plants to keep yourself safe.

Chapter 5: Turmeric

Turmeric is an Indian space that has been used for centuries in order to help us as humans to avoid illness. It is still being used today for this reason, and the ancient healing art of Ayurveda has been utilizing this particular for thousands of years. It's full of antibiotics and antioxidants, and to prevent inflammation. Bacterial, so it helps to alleviate germs that we have consumed that caused us to suffer from illnesses.

Not only that, but it's a powerful agent, one that helps to remove toxins in our bodies and get rid of any heavy metals that may have infiltrated into the bloodstream. This can prevent us from developing serious conditions down the line, and neurological disorders associated with Alzheimer's and dementia. You are worried about your health in the future, seeking out anti-inflammatory drug like turmeric is going to be the best thing that you could ever do for yourself. Turmeric is extremely healthy, and has been a healing medicinal plant for thousands of years.

Not only that, but it has also been linked to helping issues like oppression. Oppression can afflict almost anybody, and turmeric has been sworn by to help cure this mental difficulty. Discussed damage to another, whether mentally or physically, and turmeric help us to heal from both. All of us can benefit from some more of these healing medicinal plants in our lives. It can help to keep us less stressed out, which can also contribute to greater chances of healing and wellness. Stress can physically harm us, so we are able to get rid of depression and stress, these medicinal plants have even more benefits than you would think.

Chapter 6: Cardamom

Incredible healing agent as well, but also originates from India. The ancient healing art of Ayurvea this plant, and it has been used for many different things throughout the years. The body to be able to be treated by medicinal plants, such as car to mom. Cardamom can be particularly useful if you are suffering from ulcers, especially those that are in the mouth. Cardamom used to be chewed by people in order to treat and cure bad breath after meals.

Cardamom is especially useful in fighting fungus and mold, helping us to detoxify our bodies and get rid of all kinds of different problems. Mold around our house can be killed using detergents with cardamom in them, and if we are suffering from any kinds of diseases or blood clots, cardamom can help to soothe the inflammation and provide relief in this aspect. It's also an incredible helper when it comes to detoxifying the body and keeping arthritis that bay. Believe, the anti-inflammatory properties of mom are extremely powerful.

And to top it all off, cardamom can even help to cure cancer. Cancer is one of the most dangerous and scary diseases out there, and most of us are working very hard to avoid it. This may be why you have turned to medicinal plants in the first place. All of our natural chemicals going into our bodies can only be contributing to diseases down the line. Cardamom can help us to fight cancer and stay healthy for as long as possible. We are each entitled to a better way of carrying our illnesses, and one that we can trust that other people are not trying to benefit from.

Conclusion

Overall, medicinal plants are extremely beneficial and can help us to prevent being used and abused by the medicinal industry. Companies can often try to manipulate us into using experimental drugs that they claim will help us, when in reality they are actually harming us more. The chemicals we are consuming from these drugs not only harm us, they also harm the rivers and lakes in the oceans, causing deformities and marine life and difficulties and their typical way of life.

Using this beginners guide for medicinal plants, you will be able to avoid a lot of the issues that come with relying on the medicinal industry. You'll be able to help yourself and your family safer, and also to contribute to the betterment of the world at large by avoiding more unnecessary use of dangerous chemical drugs.

Everybody can benefit from more knowledge about the world around them, and if you are worried that the medicinal industry is trying to manipulate you, you probably should be. Using medicinal plants will help you to stay healthy for longer and to prevent diseases that many drugs actually cause. But don't take our word for it, try for yourself and see how much better you feel. You'll be glad you did.

Mason Jars

Discover And Learn These Top 9 Benefits Of Why You Must Include And Use Prepping Mason Jars For Any Disaster Situation Or Catastrophe

Table Of Contents

Introduction

Why I Wrote This Book

What You Should Know Before Reading This Book

Chapter 1 : Canning Food

Chapter 2 : Starting Fires

Chapter 3 : Catching Water

Chapter 4 : Keep Herbs and Spices Dry

Chapter 5 : Weapons

Chapter 6 : Storing Ammo For Other Weapons

Chapter 7 : First Aid Supplies

Chapter 8 : Store Drinks

Chapter 9 : Saving Seeds

Conclusion

Introduction

The uncertainty of our survival looms over us every day, whether we think about it or not. Anything could happen to us at any time, so it's always best to be prepared for the worst. When the best ways that you can prepare yourself for survival during a disaster catastrophe is to make sure that you have plenty of Mason jars on hand.

Having Mason jars on hand during a disaster is the best thing you can do for yourself. In this book, you're going to learn nine amazing ways that having a Mason jar during a catastrophe can benefit you and aid in your survival.

Don't wait until it's too late to learn why having Mason jars is the best thing that you could do for yourself during a catastrophe.

Why I Wrote This Book

I wrote this book because it's important to me to everybody else to survive. I'm not special when it comes to that, and neither are you. If anything happens to us, were going to try to find the best way that we can to make things work for ourselves. Whether that means having enough Mason jars, or stealing Mason jars from our friends next door, survival is as survival guide. It's better to be prepared ahead of time, so make sure that you know everything you need about Mason jars to make your life easier during a survival situation. I wrote this book so you can make it.

What You Need To Know Before Reading This Book

Before you read this book, you should remember that preparing for a survival situation has a lot of elements to it. There are more than just Mason jars when it comes to having everything you need for your survival during a catastrophe. Make sure that you are well informed and know as much as you can about preparation and disaster prevention. That's the only way that you'll be able to keep yourself and your family safe during a time of crisis. Mason jars are a great start, but there's a lot of things that you should know, so stay informed and stay safe.

Chapter 1: Canning Food

Having Mason jars is an essential piece of equipment for any survival or disaster situation. Mason jars have multiple uses, and probably the most obvious is that you can canned food in them for preservation for the long-term. It may take some knowledge and skills about how you should can your food, but once you have your system down (it mostly involves boiling acidic foods until the air is seeped out of the can until it is sealed) you'll be wondering to yourself why you haven't been preserving food for your whole life.

This is particularly useful when you don't know when your next meal may be coming, so having somewhere to store your food is extremely useful. However, Canning food isn't the only way that you can use Mason jars for food storage. There are other incredible benefits to Mason jars when it comes to survival.

Mason jars are able to keep out any unwanted pests and rodents that may be trying to get into your stock, so it only makes sense that you should use them to store all your foods. Whether they need to be preserved long-term through the canning process or you simply pour in a few cups of dry rice or beans, Mason jars keep your food safe for a long time and easy to transport in a small bag. This can be essential during a catastrophe, especially if you find yourself needing to be on the run. They pack easily into bags of any size, so you'll always have food at the ready.

Chapter 2: Starting Fires

The seasons change, depending on where you live, the more likely than not you'll probably find yourself in a cold area. Fire is what separates us from the animals in a way, and it's the thing that helps us to cook our food and find warmth and have late when we need it. Fire was the greatest invention of our ancestors, and without it, we have a very difficult time surviving in the wild. It's one of the most important things to have, and if we are in the words when it's damp and dark and can't find dry enough firewood, we can easily become ill and even die.

Fortunately, there are Mason jars that we can use to keep our fire starting supplies nice and dry. It's recommended to have kindling and tender stored away in a dry area along with matches so that you can have whatever you need to start a fire whenever possible. It's hard to catch a damp log on fire with just a small flame, and so you will have to slowly build up your fire using tinder and kindling. Having access to fire is not only a necessity for cooking raw meat, but it can also save your life. If you find yourself damp or wet, drying your clothes is a necessity.

It can also award away wildlife, and give you light if you don't have a flashlight or lantern available. Making sure that you are able to start a fire reliably during any kind of survival or disaster situation is a necessity. There are so many different uses to Mason jars, but this might just be one of the top five best ways to use a Mason jar to save your life during a catastrophe or disaster situation.

Chapter 3: Catching Water

People think about food when it comes to survival, but in reality water is what we really need to keep on hand at all times. Many people don't think about the fact that we will die after three days without water as opposed to a few weeks without food. Because of this, it's very important to make sure that you have enough water stored for yourself during any kind of disaster or survival situation. Unfortunately, that may not always be possible and so there has to be an alternative for you to try and collect water for yourself during whatever trials and tribulations you may find.

Fortunately, Mason jars serve many purposes and can also serve as a cup and a way of catching rainwater for yourself so that you can begin storing water away in your survival pantry so that you can have access to it without having to find a water source right away. Harvesting rainwater is currently just something that many environmentally conscious people do in order to save electricity that is used when we use running water. However, during a disaster, catching rainwater may just be the thing that will save our lives. If we don't have anything in which to store the water or to catch it in, we might as well be goners.

Fortunately for us, Mason jars provide us with the opportunity to provide a receptacle in which we can store water for ourselves for future use or even immediate consumption. Being able to collect water is extremely important, especially if you aren't anywhere near an available water source. Having Mason jars on hand for this, or even just to act as a water bottle during a journey through a catastrophe.

Chapter 4: Keep Herbs And Spices Dry

One thing that you need to make sure that you have during any kind of catastrophe is access to medical herbs and spices and minerals like salt that are necessary for our survival. Without salt, our bodies can become very unhealthy, so it's important to make sure that we are able to have access to these things. Not only is it useful to have medical herbs due to this high likelihood that we can catch infection during the catastrophe and injure ourselves in any number of ways, but it's also useful to make sure that these herbs are well preserved and are not invaded by pests, rodents, or rain.

Making sure that your medical herbs are kept dry and you have a place to store them as you find them out in nature is really useful. Mason jars have so many uses that it's unbelievable, and one of the most important is to make sure to keep the important things in your inventory dry and available to use. Many people don't think ahead and have airtight containers like Mason jars that they can use for long-term storage of useful items. Fortunately, Mason jars can make sure that your herbs and spices stay dry so that you don't have to suffer without them.

Making sure to have salt on hand is also extremely helpful because it can allow you to preserve meats. If you find yourself hunting for your survival, this is especially useful so that you can use all parts of a large animal that you may find and carry them along with you in a smaller and more compact way. Mason jars allow this to be easy for you and give you an area to store your food in a dry and airtight space that can't be invaded by anything except you or maybe another person.

Chapter 5: Weapons

In a pinch, you never know when you're going to need a weapon at hand. It may be because the weapon you had previously got broken or lost, or maybe you're in a survival situation involving a confrontation with something much bigger and more dangerous than yourself. Whether this is another person or a wild animal, the odds of you surviving the encounter without added help and tools may be unlikely.

Fortunately, you know that Mason jars are an extremely useful thing to have during any disaster or catastrophe. With this knowledge, you will have Mason jars on hand and thusly be able to smash the Mason jar and find a fragment glass that you can use as a weapon. Not only does this help in a pinch, such as it would help during a bar fight to break a bottle and chase after somebody, but if you're not in an emergency situation, you can use the glass shards of the Mason jar to fashion yourself an entirely new and more functioning than one that may have been previously lost or broken or nonexistent.

For this reason, it's extra-useful to have a Mason jar available. It can also help to have some kind of a grinding stone that you can use to shape a spirit or arrowhead out of glass fragments. You may want to look into making weapons prior to preparing for a disaster situation just in case you may find yourself in need of one in the future. It's better to be safe than sorry, in preparation is the entire point of this whole book.

Chapter 6: Storing Ammo For Other Weapons

People don't consider how difficult it can be to survive and a dangerous situation, and when it comes down to it, you're going to need weapons for one reason or another during the catastrophe. You may be fighting off evils of the wild or people who are trying to oppress you or attack you for one reason or another. Another reason you may need to have a way to defend yourself is that people are going to be desperate, and if they discover that you are better prepared than they are to undertake the task at hand and survive the current situation, they're going to attempt to overthrow you and usurp your resources for the assurance of their own survival.

People do desperate things during desperate times, and if they're trying to protect themselves or their families, you never know what the be capable of. There's also the option of you being out in the wilderness alone, and having to confront wild animals. If you are in a survival situation, not only are you going to need to hunt to survive in some cases, but you may not be able to defend yourself against nature. For this reason, it's very important to have Mason jars available.

You may wonder why, but using Mason jars to store ammunition for your weapons is extremely helpful. You'll be able to have easy access to them when you need them, and keep them dry and away from anybody who may attempt to be stealing them. The elements wont affect them, and nothing will invade them or try and steal them away. Keeping your ammunition safe is a very important key to survival during a catastrophe.

Chapter 7: First Aid Supplies

When it comes to a catastrophe, there is no guarantee that you going to make it out without any injuries. If you don't have a safe place to store your first aid supplies, you may end up dying of infection before you die of starvation or thirst. That would be extremely counterproductive, especially if you've done all kinds of preparation for a survival ahead of time. Fortunately, there are many first-aid kits available, and even better, if you have access to enough Mason jars, you'll be able to take these supplies with you in an easy to transport and contact form that will not be quite as flimsy as the plastic cases that they generally come in from the store.

You need to make sure that everything you have is up-to-date, at least as up-to-date as possible, and stored in a dry area where they won't be ruined. There is no point in having bandages that won't stick anymore because they've been contaminated by some kind of moisture. The same is true of gauze and healing ointments. If they are infiltrated in any way, it can be very dangerous for your help during an emergency.

Keeping your emergency first aid supplies and a Mason jar is also useful because you have tubes of appointment, they can often burst under the pressure applied under your weight or in the mix and crannies of a disorganized backpack. Keeping it in a glass Mason jar is a great idea because it will make sure to preserve your precious supplies for when they are needed the most.

Chapter 8: Storing Drinks

Some may argue with this, but often times one of the only highlights of being in a disaster or survival situation is being able to have a drink every once in a while. Although it's not recommended to drink regularly, if you are in a survival situation and you find yourself in the unique position to brew some sort of ale to help you get yourself through the day more easily, having Mason jars to store your drinks and is way to travel with them after making a batch to store them for further usage in the future.

Although it is recommended to John your problems with alcohol, especially because you're not going to want to be foggy minded during a survival situation, it can prove as useful bartering tools if you discover that you need supplies of some sort but aren't sure how or where to get them.

It's always better to be clearheaded during a survival, and it's well known that junk people don't with a very high efficiency. It may be the fastest way to get yourself killed, then again, it may be the only way to help you get through it until the end. You might as well have enough Mason jars on hand that you can store your brew and keep it fresh for as long as possible.

Chapter 9: Saving Seeds

It is impossible to say what may happen during the specific catastrophe or survival situation you may find yourself in during the future. However, if you plan to have any type of long-term survival if society happened to collapse and you're having a difficult time moving forward, something you're really going to want to have on your side in terms of the future are seedlings.

A survival situation is going to be tough, but it's going to be tougher if it's long-term. You can find a place where you can survive safely and maybe you can settle down long enough to start and trying get society back on track. If your community has been ravaged by some sort of terrible problem, at least that you should be doing is trying to create a more sustainable way of life.

If a food shortage is part of the catastrophe, having a Mason jar to store seeds and so that you can plant them later on and have food security for the rest of your life is essential. You need to keep them in a dry and safe place, so Mason jars are ideal. They keep out the water and they keep out unwanted pasts that may try and eat them or steal them. If you want to think about the future, you should have a Mason jar.

Conclusion

Overall, surviving is a lot of work. But it's worth it can be done easily using the aid of Mason jars. If you have enough Mason jars, you'll be able to have so many advantages over other people who might be in a similar situation. Having a Mason jar available can often save your life, and it's simply a matter of time out in the wild before you will see all the uses of a Mason jar for yourself. Make sure you are prepared right now for what may happen in the future and get yourself a bunch of these amazing jars to aid in your survival today!

Lose Weight

Discover The Beginners Guide To Learning How You Can Lose Weight And Burn Fat EASILY!

Table Of Contents

Introduction

Why I Wrote This Book

What You Should Know Before Reading This Book

Chapter 1 : Changing Your Diet

Chapter 2 : Maintaining A Regular Exercise Routine

Chapter 3 : Support Circle

Chapter 4 : Positive Thinking

Chapter 5 : Dangers Of Trend Diets

Chapter 6 : Tips and Tricks

Conclusion

Introduction

Most of us have wanted to lose weight at one time or another. It is difficult to consider our lives without the constant goal of losing a few pounds or looking a little better in this way or that. We have many different ideals for ourselves, and even if we are at our ideal weight, there are other ways that we would like to begin to tone our bodies and become closer to the image we envision for ourselves. Many people have a difficult time becoming comfortable with a routine that works for them, and this book is here to help!

What holds us back from losing weight? There are so many things, and only by addressing them will we be able to fully embrace the people we want to become and bridge the gap between us now and who we will become in the future. We have to know it is possible, believe it, and see the steps clearly so that we can take them and get the results we desire. Who doesn't want to look a little better, be a little healthier? Who wouldn't want to do this quickly and effectively? That is a goal each and every one of us could get behind, and this is the book to help you to launch over your fears and help you become the person of your dreams.

Whether you want to lose over 300 pounds or you would like to tone your body to the desired state, this book will have advice for you. Everybody works at their own pace, and comparing yourself to other people and their progress in their unique journeys is the first step in self-defeat and unhappiness. If you really want to lose weight, keep it off, and maintain a healthy lifestyle, reading this book will show you what to do to accomplish your weight-loss goals quickly and easily, and in a way that will benefit you in the future and for the rest of your life!

Why I Wrote This Book

I wrote this book because I know what it is like to be stuck in a rut. Many people have a difficult time losing weight and being their ideal size. All of us have looked in the mirror before and wondered what in the world we are doing wrong. The truth is that we simply do not have thee right amount of confidence to pursue this weight loss as a lifestyle rather than a small isolated effort. This can be dangerous, because maintaining a healthy lifestyle is the only way to really indulge in the long-term benefits and goals that we set for ourselves.

Getting discouraged because we don't get immediate results is a terrible thing, because changing your life is often not an over-night process. It takes a whole re-wiring of your mindset before you can do so, and we should never compare our progress to that of other people. The only time this is okay is if it is in a consentually competitive way, to help one another along. It should never be a way to measure yourself up or guage your worth. As long as you get up every day and try, you are doing just as well as everybody else. Many people never even get that far, so you should be proud!

I wrote this book because I am tired of the world fat-shaming people and telling them they are not working hard enough. Chances are, we have gained weight for reasons beyond our control and since then have just spiralled out of control. Whether the origin is in bad eating habits, depression, lack of self-esteem, physical disorders, pregnancy, or any other very reasonable cause of weight gain, chances are we want to lose the weight and be healthier. The issue here remains that people should never be shamed for their body type, whether they are a thousand pounds or not. Especially if they are doing their best to help themselves to live a strong and independent life where they work to be the person they want to be.

I want to help you to understand the nature of weight loss, help you have a positive view of yourself, and make changes in your life that are easy and will help you become the person you have always wanted to be. That is the reason why I wrote this book.

What You Need To Know Before Reading This Book

Before you read this book it is important to keep in mind that not every diet plan you may follow will have your best interest in mind. Most of these diets are built so that people have to pay for extra information that has been hyped up and makes wild claims to help us to lose weight quickly and easily. The fact is that losing weight quickly can be very dangerous, and many of these diets rely on methods that put our bodies into starvation mode and eat away at our muscles, which makes it even harder to prevent weight gain in the future and can cause us to gain weight rapidly because we have no muscles working for us to burn the fat we consume.

Low carb diets can be especially dangerous, as they force the body to seek alternative sources of energy. If it cannot find carbs to use for energy, the ideal of most low carb diets is that it will seek to find our excess fat stores and use those up for energy rather than our muscles. However, there is no guarantee that the body will not use our muscles first. In fact, it may very well go there first because it is a higher protein source of energy. These can leave us sick and more vulnerable to weight fluctuations in the future that become harder and harder to avoid and battle in a healthy way.

For this reason, it is important to make sure you lose weight the right way. The right way may not seem as fast, but it is just as easy, if not more so! You will be astounded by the way your body and life can change with the right determination and dedication to the right regime, and what they don't seem to want you to know is that the best method to losing weight doesn't have to do with altering your body's chemistry. What it really relies on is making conscious choices about what you eat and how you eat it and maintaining good habits.

Creating good habits can start right now! Don't let these dangerous fad diets lure you in with false promises. You deserve better than that, and should always be skeptical of manipulative promises that will end up hurting you and costing you unforseen amounts of money and going back on its promise. Much of the time you will lose pounds fast enough that you will spread the word of these horrible diets, only to discover that it stops working after a certain point and you are gaining weight again and having an even harder time losing it this time. I want to make sure you are doing things right so you can be happy and satisfied with the results!

Chapter 1: Changing Your Diet

One of the easiest ways you can lose weight quickly is by changing your diet. Although many people will swear by low-carb diets, the fact remains that you are unlikely to physically maintain such a diet for long, and they can be completely devastating to your body. What really works is even easier than spending hours counting calories and figuring out whether or not you can have a carbohydrate cheat day in order to prevent your body from shutting down and going into starvation mode. What actually helps is changing your diet.

If you were to eat foods that were lower in starches and sugars, and turn to foods that are free of toxins and chemical pesticides, like organic fruits and vegetables and lean, hormone and antibiotic free meats and poultry, it will make it easier for your body to let go of your fat. Toxins in the body actually bind fat to them and stick around a lot longer, so going through a detox can often cause us to lose weight quickly and effectively without gaining it all back right away. We are able to fully utilize the body's natural systems to help us to balance ourselves back out by avoiding the foods that are bad for us and helping our bodies to eliminate them.

Some great foods that can help us to get rid of toxins and act as antioxidants are green tea, aloe vera gel, many Indian spices like turmeric and curry, and blackberries and blueberries. These help us to get rid of toxins and keep our bodies healthy for the long term. It is also really important to make sure that you are drinking a lot of water because water can help to ensure that our livers and kidneys are working properly to flush toxins out of the body so they are not stuck inside of us and trapping fat.

Chapter 2: Maintaining A Regular Exercise Routine

Another important aspect of losing weight is maintaining a regular exercise routine. Nobody can have weight loss and maintain it properly without having enough exercise. It is inevitable that we will just go right back to where we started if we don't begin to seek ways to keep our bodies strong and continue to lose weight. It is just the sad truth of things. Fortunately, there are a lot of ways for us to get exercise without feeling as if it is a huge hassle. Something as simple as getting up and taking a walk every day is a great way to help us to burn fat and feel great. And even if you never envisioned yourself heading to the gym, that can be for the best, considering many people can injure themselves if they do not exercise properly.

If you do want to try the gym out, the best thing you can do to lose weight fast and easily is to work with a personal trainer who knows and understands your personal challenges and the needs of your body. It can be difficult to use equipment properly and many people injure themselves, so it is a great idea to learn from somebody who understands your unique situation. It can also be beneficial to have a personal trainer because they hold you accountable to your actions and diet and continue to motivate you to continue to succeed, no matter what.

Regular exercise is extremely beneficial to weight loss for another reason. Our muscles are the main way that our bodies are able to burn fat quickly. If we are not spending time building our muscles, then our fat will settle in our bodies easily because there is nothing there telling it that it shouldn't. Our muscles aren't able to burn as many calories and we find ourselves gaining weight fast because we aren't doing what we need to be doing to stay healthy. Everybody should have at least half an hour of exercise three times per week, even if that simply means getting up and taking a walk!

Chapter 3: Support Circle

Something most people overlook when they are trying to lose weight is the benefit of finding a great support circle. A support circle could be just you and one friend or yourself and a whole group of people who you trust with your personal struggles and challenges. These people will be there to help you through the thick and the thin, and you will be there to help them as well. As long as it is a healthy and constructive environment, you will be more motivated to keep yourself on track and continue working hard toward your goals.

Many people find support circles beneficial toward their personal weight-loss goals because of its accountability factor. Many of us have a difficult time being realistic about our actions and how they affect the results that we want. Many times we don't realize what we are doing that can sabotage our efforts, and having a group to share our struggles with can force us to face up to the truth about ourselves.

This can be majorly important for people who have struggled with losing weight in the past, and can jump start a routine that can help you maintain a lifelong weight loss goal for the rest of your days. It is an amazing way to really get yourself on the fast track to success!

Chapter 4: Power Of Positive Thinking

The sad truth about weight gain is that much of it can come as a way of coping with negative thoughts and experiences. Sometimes our excess weight can show an even bigger problem just under the surface. If this is the case, positive thinking can play a bigger role than you think in jump starting your weight loss adventure today.

Sometimes, therapy can be an effective tool in weight loss. It can help us get to the root of the problem, such as why we may not feel we deserve to have a healthy body, or to get over the hurdles that depression can place in front of us as we attempt to work our way toward a better future. Whatever you decide to use to help you think more positively, the results will be profound and you will discover yourself feeling better than ever, and more motivated to do right by yourself and your body!

Positive thinking can physically change us, and can change our outlook on life. It has been proven to reduce stress and help us to see the silver lining when things look impossible. Many people who struggle with weight loss have a tendency to believe it is going to be impossible to change their lives. Fortunately, it is both possible and easy to do so by making just a few simple changes in your life!

Chapter 5: The Dangers Of Fad Diets

If your main goal is to lose weight, using a fad diet is not the way to do it. Chances are, the more popular diets are scams that will ultimately harm your body far more than they will help it. Most trendy diets can lead to serious health problems and increased weight gain later in life.

They promise to help us lose weight by changing something in our body's chemistry. They use scientific jargon to convince us to starve ourselves with low carb diets or other dangerous things, like the HCG hormone, claiming we can cheat the system by doing something dangerous, like injecting hormones or putting our bodies into starvation mode to shed a few pounds of muscle.

Unfortunately, these diets can never be maintained long term without serious health consequences and most of them cause excessive weight gain. Every pound you lost from that diet will come back with a vengeance and be harder to lose. This is because they generally begin to harm our muscle mass, which is responsible for all of the healthy fat burning that takes place within the body. It is very dangerous to try to do things the fast and easy way using a fad or trend diet. Instead, work hard on building muscles that will burn your fat and get plenty of rest and exercise.

Chapter 6: Tips and Tricks

If you want some tips and tricks for fast weight loss, try going vegan. This is a drastic diet that cuts out a lot of sources of fat intake, and many people find themselves undergoing a drastic change in body weight as they proceed on a vegan diet. Not only that, but it's great for the environment and the animals you are choosing not to eat!

Another thing that helps is having a good work out soundtrack that gets you excited to move your body and change your life. Sometimes exercise can be very easy and fun. Things like swimming and dancing can be great weight loss activities that help people who have a difficult time enjoying gym equipment to have fun losing weight. Swimming is particularly helpful if you have any body injuries that you need to be careful of as you exercise.

Eating things like grapefruit and cooking coconut oil can also aid in weight loss without having to do much else. Cabbage is another food that helps the body to lose weight more rapidly.

Another important thing to keep in mind is to stop feeling like you are changing your diet and can not eat certain foods. Change "Can not" to "should not," but give yourself permission to make your own choices. This will take a lot of pressure off and relieve the stress and guilt you may feel from making poor dietary choices, leaving you comfortable enough to say to yourself, "I may not have done well today but I will do better tomorrow," and mean it.

Conclusion

Overall, losing weight quickly and easily is a goal for everybody. We can all lose weight according to our own terms – we just have to figure out how to set them! Using the tips in this book, everybody should be able to figure out which particular stragegy might work for them and utilize it to change their lives!

We can all relate to wanting to lose weight, here or there in our lives. Everything that we do can affect us in the future, and if you really want to stay healthy, the key is in prevention. Don't allow yourself to lose sight of your end goal – always keep the future you in mind and never let go of your dreams! You'll be so glad you didn't. Use this beginners guide to help yourself achieve your goals and change your life today!